Life Without Gluten

The Good, the Bad, and the Delicious Without All the Glute!

Katherine McGuire

Table of Contents

Introduction

Welcome to the gluten-free world, where the journey of celiac disease and gluten sensitivity begins. In this book, we will embark on a comprehensive exploration of the fascinating world of gluten-related disorders, debunking myths and shedding light on the truth behind gluten-free living. So, fasten your seatbelts and get ready for an eye-opening adventure that will change the way you perceive gluten forever.

Imagine a world where a seemingly innocent protein, gluten, holds the power to wreak havoc on the human body. Celiac disease, a complex autoimmune disorder, takes center stage in this intricate tale. We'll look into the depths of this condition, examining its causes, symptoms, and the impact it has on the lives of those affected. Brace yourself as we navigate through the maze of celiac disease, uncovering its enigmatic nature and the challenges faced by those living with it.

Gluten-sensitive enteropathy, another name for celiac disease, is not just an intolerance or a preference in diet, but is a significant immunological disorder that is brought on by dietary consumption. Gluten is a protein included in wheat, barley, and rye. When individuals with celiac disease consume gluten, their immune system responds by attacking the small intestine, leading to inflammation and damage to the delicate villi that line the intestinal walls. The consequences can be far-reaching, affecting not only the digestive system but also various other organs and systems in the body.

But wait, there's more to the story. Gluten sensitivity, often overshadowed by celiac disease, demands our attention. While it does not involve the same autoimmune response as celiac disease, gluten sensitivity can still cause significant discomfort and adverse reactions in individuals who are sensitive to gluten. Symptoms such as bloating, abdominal pain, fatigue, and headaches can arise after gluten consumption, prompting individuals to seek answers and explore a gluten-free lifestyle.

To comprehend the gluten-free world fully, you must first understand its antagonist: gluten. We will embark on a scientific expedition into the fascinating world of this perplexing protein. From its origins in wheat and other grains to its composition and structure, we'll dissect gluten molecule by molecule, unraveling its secrets along the way. We'll explore the unique properties of gluten that make it both a culinary delight and a potential health hazard for those with gluten-related disorders.

What happens when gluten enters the body? Prepare to venture into the intricate interactions between gluten and the immune system, unraveling the mechanisms behind the body's immune response in celiac disease and gluten sensitivity. Through captivating anecdotes and expert insights, we'll shed light on the mysterious dance between gluten and the human body. We'll explore the genetic factors that contribute to the development of celiac disease, as well as the role of environmental triggers in activating the immune response.

Gluten-related disorders have been making headlines, leaving many to wonder about their prevalence in today's society. We will also embark on a statistical expedition, uncovering the prevalence of celiac disease and gluten sensitivity across different populations and regions. We'll look at what's causing these problems to become more prevalent, as well as the effects they have on general health. From the increasing awareness of gluten-related disorders to the challenges of accurate diagnoses, we'll navigate through the complex landscape of gluten-related disorders in the modern world.

But how do these disorders affect individuals on a personal level? Through touching personal stories, we'll hear the voices of those living with celiac disease and gluten sensitivity. Their experiences will shed light on the challenges they face, the impact on their daily lives, and the resilience that fuels their determination to thrive in a gluten-filled world. From navigating social gatherings and dining out, to finding gluten-free alternatives and dealing with the emotional aspects of living with a chronic condition, their stories will inspire and provide insights into the realities of gluten-related disorders.

As we learn more about living a gluten-free lifestyle, we come across a web of untruths and misconceptions about conditions that are linked to gluten. Brace yourself as we embark on a myth-busting expedition, debunking popular beliefs that cloud our understanding of celiac disease and gluten sensitivity. From the myth of gluten sensitivity being a trendy fad, to the notion that a gluten-free diet is a weight-loss miracle, we'll expose the truth behind these misconceptions. Armed with scientific evidence and expert opinions, we'll navigate through the sea of misinformation, empowering you with the knowledge needed to make informed decisions about your health.

As we conclude our exploration of the gluten-free world, we hope you will gain a fresh perspective on celiac disease, gluten sensitivity, and the intricacies of gluten-related disorders. By arming yourself with this newfound understanding, you can navigate the challenges of gluten-free living with confidence and grace. Whether you have been diagnosed with celiac disease or gluten sensitivity, or simply want to learn more about this captivating subject, this book serves as your guide, offering valuable insights, practical tips, and a sense of community.

Keep in mind that you are not journeying alone. Along the way, we've shared stories of triumph, dispelled myths, and delved into the science behind gluten-related disorders. By embracing the gluten-free world, you join a vibrant community of individuals who strive for health and happiness despite the obstacles. Together, we can challenge the status quo, promote awareness, and create a world where gluten-related disorders are understood and accommodated.

So, as you turn the page and embark on the chapters that lie ahead, be prepared for a transformative experience. The gluten-free world awaits, ready to challenge your preconceptions, ignite your curiosity, and empower you to embrace a life free from the shackles of gluten.

Chapter 1:

The Gluten-Free Lifestyle

Unveiled

Are you ready to love and embrace the gluten-free lifestyle? In this chapter, we will explore the essential aspects of the gluten-free lifestyle, providing insights, tips, and tricks to navigate the gluten-free world with confidence. From embracing a gluten-free mindset to mastering grocery shopping, stocking your pantry, and dining out or traveling gluten-free, we will cover all the important aspects to help you adopt and thrive in the gluten-free lifestyle.

Embracing a Gluten-Free Mindset: Challenges and Opportunities

The gluten-free market's significant growth, with a projected compound annual growth rate of 9.8% from 2022 to 2030 ("2023 Trends," 2023), is a testament to the increasing prevalence of gluten-related disorders and the rising demand for gluten-free products by consumers. This growth has led to exciting opportunities for individuals embracing a gluten-free lifestyle. It does, however, also have its share of difficulties.

One of the main challenges in gluten-free product development is dough handling. Gluten-free dough and batters lack the viscosity and elasticity of their gluten-containing counterparts, which can make them difficult to process and machine. For baked goods and other gluten-free items, the lack of gluten presents particular difficulties in producing the correct texture and structure. However, these challenges have spurred the food industry to continuously adapt and improve formulations and processing techniques to meet consumer expectations.

It is important to recognize that the primary role of the gluten-free diet is to manage gluten-related disorders such as celiac disease, gluten sensitivity, and wheat allergies. For individuals with these conditions, following a gluten-free diet is essential to preventing adverse health effects. The widespread usage of a gluten-free diet for nonmedical reasons, however, is not supported by a lot of scientific evidence. While some individuals may choose a gluten-free lifestyle for personal reasons, it is crucial to be mindful of the potential limitations and nutritional inadequacies associated with this dietary approach.

The sensory limitations of gluten-free products have been a common concern among individuals adopting a gluten-free lifestyle. Texture, taste, and mouthfeel are important factors in the overall enjoyment of food, and gluten-free products may not always match the sensory experiences of their gluten-containing counterparts.

However, significant efforts have been made to improve the sensory attributes of gluten-free products with advancements in ingredient technology and formulation techniques. Consumers can now find a wide range of gluten-free products that closely resemble their gluten-containing counterparts in taste and texture.

Another challenge faced by individuals embracing a gluten-free lifestyle is ensuring a nutritionally balanced diet. The removal of gluten-containing grains such as wheat, barley, and rye may impact the intake of certain nutrients such as fiber, B vitamins, and iron. However, there are many naturally gluten-free grains and other nutrient-dense alternatives available to maintain a well-rounded diet. You can satisfy your nutritional needs by consuming a range of gluten-free whole grains, fruits, vegetables, lean proteins, and dairy products.

Navigating Grocery Shopping for Gluten-Free Products

Navigating grocery shopping for gluten-free products can initially seem overwhelming, but with the right knowledge and guidance, it becomes easier over time. Searching for the Gluten-Free Certification Program (GFCP) label on products is an essential consideration. This certification ensures that the products meet strict standards for gluten-free labeling, providing you with confidence and peace of mind while shopping. When you see the GFCP logo on packaging, you can trust that the product has undergone thorough testing and meets the necessary criteria to be labeled gluten-free.

Reading food labels becomes a crucial skill for identifying gluten-free products. Initially, label reading might feel daunting, but with practice, it becomes more comfortable and efficient. Look for keywords like "gluten-free," "certified gluten-free," or "made in a dedicated gluten-free facility" on the packaging. These labels indicate that the product has been specifically manufactured and handled to prevent cross-contamination with gluten-containing ingredients.

Learn about frequent places where gluten is hidden to improve your ability to read food labels. Some ingredients that may contain gluten include malt, modified food starch, and certain flavorings. By knowing which ingredients to watch out for, you can make informed decisions about the products you choose to purchase. Additionally, be aware that some products may have a "may contain" statement, indicating potential cross-contamination, even if the ingredients themselves are gluten-free. When deciding if you want to buy these things, use your discretion and degree of comfort.

Navigating the grocery store can be simplified by asking customer service for guidance and information on gluten-free product locations. Some stores even have dedicated gluten-free aisles, making it convenient for you to find a wide range of gluten-free options in one place (Nardone, n.d.). However, not all stores have dedicated aisles, so it's essential to explore different sections of the store. Remember that many naturally gluten-free foods are found on the perimeter, such as fruits, vegetables, seafood, meats, and dairy. Incorporating these whole, unprocessed foods into your diet is a healthy and gluten-free choice.

Connecting with nearby support groups or online forums that concentrate on gluten-free living is another useful suggestion. These groups frequently promote gluten-free goods, companies, and shops in your neighborhood. They can offer insightful advice to improve the effectiveness and pleasure of your grocery shopping.

By following these tips and arming yourself with knowledge about gluten-free certification, label reading, and store navigation, you can confidently navigate grocery shopping for gluten-free products. Over time, you'll become more familiar with brands and products that suit your dietary needs, making the process feel much less overwhelming.

Stocking Your Pantry With Essential Gluten-Free Ingredients

To embark on a successful gluten-free cooking journey, it's essential to have a well-stocked pantry filled with key ingredients that cater to your dietary needs. Here are some must-have gluten-free pantry essentials that will empower you to create delicious and satisfying meals at home:

- **Gluten-free all-purpose flour:** A reliable gluten-free all-purpose flour blend is a game-changer in gluten-free cooking. It offers a simple replacement for conventional wheat flour in numerous recipes, saving time and effort. Whether you're making pancakes, muffins, or pizza dough, a high-quality commercial all-purpose blend will mimic the texture and performance of wheat flour, allowing you to achieve excellent results.

- **White and brown rice flour:** Rice flour is a versatile staple in gluten-free baking. Due to its mild flavor and light texture, it can be used in a variety of cuisines. White rice flour is ideal for delicate cakes, cookies, and pastries, while brown rice flour adds a nutty flavor and extra fiber to baked goods. To achieve the right texture and flavor, these flours can be used alone or in conjunction with other gluten-free flours.

- **Gluten-free breadcrumbs:** Breadcrumbs are a handy ingredient for adding texture and flavor to dishes like breaded chicken or fish. While gluten-free breadcrumbs can be found in some supermarkets and health food stores, it's easy to make your own at home by grinding gluten-free bread or using alternative options like crushed gluten-free cereal or ground nuts. To alter the flavor profile of your breadcrumbs, try experimenting with various herbs and spices.

- **Gluten-free soy sauce and tamari:** Adding depth and complexity to your dishes is made easy with gluten-free soy sauce and tamari. These savory sauces are essential for creating flavorful stir-fries, marinades, and dressings. The best soy sauce to use is one that is expressly marked as gluten-free because traditional soy sauce frequently contains wheat. Tamari, on the other hand, is a Japanese soy sauce that is often naturally gluten-free. Check the labels to ensure they are gluten-free, and enjoy the umami-rich flavors they bring to your cooking.

- **Gluten-free pasta:** Having gluten-free pasta in your pantry opens up a world of meal possibilities. Whether you're craving a comforting bowl of spaghetti or a quick and easy pasta salad, gluten-free pasta options made from grains like corn, rice, or quinoa offer a satisfying substitute. These alternatives have come a long way in terms of taste and texture, and many brands now offer gluten-free pasta that rivals its traditional counterpart. Experiment with different shapes and varieties to find your favorites and enjoy a satisfying pasta experience without the gluten.

By stocking your pantry with these essential gluten-free ingredients, you'll have the foundation to create a wide range of flavorful dishes that cater to your dietary needs. Experiment with different recipes, incorporating these ingredients into your cooking repertoire, and discover the joy of gluten-free culinary adventures.

Tips and Tricks for Dining Out and Traveling Gluten-Free

Dining out and traveling can present challenges for individuals following a gluten-free diet, but with some careful planning and proactive measures, it's possible to enjoy meals outside of your home without anxiety. Here are some pointers and advice for traveling and eating out while avoiding gluten ("Restaurant Dining," 2019):

1. **Choose the right kind of eating establishment:** The type of restaurant you choose can greatly influence your success at gluten-free dining. Opt for restaurants that have a reputation for accommodating special dietary needs or that offer dedicated gluten-free menus. Such businesses have a greater probability to be knowledgeable about cross-contamination dangers and gluten-free preparations. Prioritize places that prioritize gluten-free practices and have positive reviews from the gluten-free community.

2. **Call ahead:** Make a reservation by calling the restaurant the day before or early on the same day to ensure a flawless eating experience. Speaking to the chef or manager allows you to discuss your dietary restrictions and meal options in advance. Inform them about your gluten-free needs, including any specific ingredients or cooking methods to avoid. This proactive

approach enables the restaurant staff to prepare in advance and accommodate your needs.

3. **Dine early or late:** You can improve your chances of getting the correct attention from the personnel by timing your meal either before or after the busiest mealtime. During peak hours, restaurants may be more rushed and less able to accommodate specific dietary requirements. By opting for off-peak dining times, such as early lunch or late dinner, you can enhance your dining experience and reduce the risk of cross-contamination.

4. **Clearly explain your dietary restrictions:** Spend some time explaining your gluten-free requirements to the wait staff before placing your order at a restaurant. Communicate your dietary limitations in plain, clear terms, emphasizing the significance of avoiding all gluten contact. It can be helpful to mention that you have celiac disease or a gluten sensitivity, as it conveys the severity of the condition. Request that your meal be prepared separately, using clean utensils and avoiding cross-contamination with gluten-containing ingredients.

5. **Clean cutlery at all times:** Forks and surfaces should be clean when preparing your food, therefore request this. Ask the restaurant about their preparation methods and if they have previously cooked any breaded or gluten-containing items on the same surface. You may lessen the chance of cross-contamination and assure the safety of your gluten-free meal by

asking for a clean surface and utensils. If necessary, emphasize the importance of separate handling and cooking to avoid any traces of gluten.

By following these tips and tricks, you can confidently navigate dining out and traveling while maintaining a gluten-free diet. Remember to communicate your needs clearly, be proactive, and advocate for yourself to ensure a safe and enjoyable dining experience.

Chapter 2

Living Well, Gluten-Free

Living a gluten-free lifestyle goes beyond just eliminating gluten from your diet. In this chapter, we will explore how to craft a well-balanced gluten-free diet, discover alternative grains and flours that can enhance your culinary experiences, delve into innovative cooking and baking techniques, and learn to identify hidden sources of gluten in unexpected foods and products. By embracing these practices, you can not only meet your dietary needs, but also enjoy delicious and satisfying gluten-free meals with a touch of creativity.

Crafting a Well-Balanced Gluten-Free Diet

Maintaining a well-balanced diet is essential for anyone, including those following a gluten-free lifestyle. It's not just about avoiding gluten; it's about nourishing your body with the right nutrients and finding joy in the foods you eat. Here are some tips for crafting a well-balanced gluten-free diet:

1. Eat regular meals based on starchy carbohydrates. Starchy carbohydrates like rice, potatoes, quinoa, and gluten-free pasta should form the foundation of your meals. These provide energy, fiber, and important nutrients. Experiment with different grains and gluten-free alternatives to keep your meals interesting and varied.

2. Set a daily goal of five servings of fruit and vegetables. In addition to providing a wealth of vitamins, minerals, and antioxidants, fruits and vegetables are naturally gluten-free. To your meal, they bring color, flavor, and nourishment. Try incorporating a rainbow of fruits and vegetables to ensure you get a diverse range of nutrients.

3. Monitor your fat intake, especially saturated fats. While fats are an important part of a balanced diet, it's crucial to choose healthy fats. Choose sources like olive oil, almonds, seeds, and avocados. Reduce your consumption of processed foods, fried foods, and fatty meats that are high in saturated fat.

4. Keep an eye on sugar. Sugar is often added to gluten-free sweets, biscuits, cakes, and full-sugar fizzy drinks to enhance flavor. Consuming too much sugar can cause a number of health problems. Opt for naturally sweetened options or make your own gluten-free treats using alternative sweeteners like honey, maple syrup, or stevia.

5. Eat plenty of fiber. Constipation can be avoided and a healthy digestive tract maintained with fiber. Consume foods high in fiber, such as fruits, vegetables, whole grains made without gluten, and legumes. Additionally, these foods give you a feeling of fullness and aid with blood sugar regulation.

6. Cut down on salt. Consuming too much salt might increase your chances of developing high blood pressure and other health issues. Processed gluten-free foods should be avoided because they sometimes have increased salt content. Use herbs, spices, and other flavorings to season your food instead of using too much salt.

Let's take a look at a story about Emma's pizza dough disaster as an example. Emma, a self-proclaimed gluten-free food enthusiast, decided to try her hand at making homemade gluten-free pizza. Armed with a new recipe and a positive attitude, she embarked on her culinary adventure.

As Emma mixed the gluten-free flour blend, added the yeast, and kneaded the dough, she couldn't help but feel a sense of accomplishment. However, when it came time to roll out the dough, things took a comical turn. The gluten-free dough seemed to have a mind of its own, resisting her attempts to shape it into a perfect circle.

Undeterred, Emma embraced the unpredictability and the misshapen form of her pizza crust. She jokingly referred to it as a gluten-free masterpiece with a unique personality. When she finally took a bite, she was pleasantly surprised by the delicious flavor and texture of her homemade creation.

The pizza dough disaster taught Emma the importance of embracing imperfection and finding joy in the process rather than striving for perfection. It became a cherished memory that she shared with friends, laughing about the unconventional shape and savoring the delicious taste of her gluten-free pizza.

Exploring Alternative Grains and Flours: Your Culinary Allies

Exploring alternative grains and flours opens up a world of culinary possibilities for those following a gluten-free diet. These ingredients not only provide unique flavors and textures, but also offer a range of nutritional benefits. Let's explore each of these gluten-free allies in more detail:

Amaranth: The extraordinary nutritional profile of this historic grain, which was once a mainstay of the Aztecs, is helping it gain appeal. Amaranth is a complete protein, meaning it contains all the essential amino acids. It is also rich in fiber, calcium, iron, and magnesium. Its slightly nutty flavor and crunchy texture make it a versatile ingredient. You can use cooked amaranth as a base for salads, blend it into porridge or soups, or even add it to gluten-free bread recipes for a delightful crunch.

Rice: One of the most popular grains in the world and a key component of gluten-free diets is rice. It comes in various types, including short-grain, long-grain, jasmine, and basmati, each with its own unique characteristics. Rice is a good source of energy and provides essential minerals like magnesium and selenium. Due to its bland flavor, it goes well with a variety of foods. Use it as a side dish, in stir-fries, as a filling for sushi rolls, or even in comforting rice pudding for a satisfying dessert.

Buckwheat: Buckwheat is naturally gluten-free, despite its name, and is not a type of wheat. In reality, it is a seed related to rhubarb and sorrel. B vitamins, fiber, and minerals like iron and magnesium are all found in abundance in buckwheat. Buckwheat flour, with its distinct flavor, can be used to make fluffy gluten-free pancakes, delicate crepes, and hearty buckwheat noodles known as soba. It gives baked items and savory foods alike a nutty flavor and distinctive texture.

Cornmeal, polenta, grits, and hominy: These gluten-free alternatives are derived from corn and provide a hearty and comforting element to meals. Cornmeal, which comes in different textures, can be used to make gluten-free cornbread, corn muffins, or corn tortillas. Polenta is a coarser version of cornmeal and can be cooked into a creamy porridge or used as a base for various toppings like sautéed mushrooms or grilled vegetables. Grits are made from ground corn and are popular in Southern cuisine, often served as a side dish for breakfast or accompanied by shrimp as a savory meal. Hominy is a type of corn that has been soaked in an alkali solution, resulting in a unique texture and flavor. Foods like the traditional Mexican soup pozole can be prepared using it.

When exploring alternative grains and flours, it's important to keep in mind that not every culinary experiment will turn out perfectly. The process of discovering new gluten-free alternatives can be filled with both successes and occasional mishaps. Embrace the humorous side of cooking, learn from any mistakes, and appreciate the journey of finding delightful gluten-free options that suit your tastes and dietary needs.

Incorporating these alternative grains and flours into your gluten-free diet not only expands your culinary repertoire, but also provides a range of nutrients and flavors. Whether you're enjoying the nutty crunch of amaranth, the versatility of rice, the distinctive taste of buckwheat, or the comforting textures of cornmeal, polenta, grits, and hominy, these gluten-free allies are here to enhance your dining experiences. So, be bold, experiment with different recipes, and savor the joy of exploring the world of gluten-free grains and flours.

Innovative Cooking and Baking Techniques for Gluten-Free Goodness

Baking and cooking gluten-free call for a different strategy than conventional techniques. However, you can produce tasty and fulfilling outcomes with a little imagination and the appropriate methods. Here are some innovative cooking and baking techniques to elevate your gluten-free culinary endeavors:

Create your own custom flour or flour and ground nut mixture: One of the joys of gluten-free baking is the freedom to experiment with different flours and create unique flavor profiles. Combine flours like sorghum, tapioca, and brown rice to develop your own versatile blend. Incorporate ground nuts, such as almonds or hazelnuts, for added richness and texture in your baked goods.

Adding xanthan gum for better texture: Gluten provides elasticity and structure to baked goods, which can be lacking in gluten-free alternatives. Adding a small amount of xanthan gum to your recipes helps mimic the qualities of gluten, resulting in less crumbly and more cohesive baked goods. Just keep in mind that less is more.

Be mindful of liquid content: Gluten-free flours tend to absorb more liquid than their gluten-containing counterparts. To prevent dryness in your baked goods, consider adding slightly more liquid than stated in the recipe. Your finished product will be delicious and moist as a result.

Adjust baking time: Due to the differences in ingredients and moisture content, gluten-free baked goods may require a slightly longer baking time. Keep an eye on your creations and extend the baking time by 5–10 minutes if needed. The ideal texture will be achieved, and any raw centers will be avoided.

Unveiling Hidden Sources of Gluten in Unexpected Foods and Products

Being gluten-free means being vigilant and aware of hidden sources of gluten that can sneak into your diet. While you may think you've eliminated gluten entirely, it can still hide in unexpected places. Here are some examples of hidden sources of gluten to keep in mind:

1. Medications and supplements: Gluten may be used as a filler or coating in medications and supplements. To make sure they are gluten-free, it is crucial to carefully examine the labels or seek advice from a medical practitioner.

2. Meat, fish, and poultry: While meat, fish, and poultry are naturally gluten-free, watch out for hydrolyzed wheat protein in processed or flavored versions. It's always best to choose fresh, unprocessed meats or check the labels of packaged products to ensure they are gluten-free.

3. Oats: Oats can be contaminated with wheat during the growing or processing stages, so it's crucial to look for certified gluten-free oats or opt for gluten-free alternatives like quinoa flakes or buckwheat groats.

4. Beverages and alcohol: Malt vinegar, commonly used in dressings and condiments, is fermented and made from barley. Chinese black vinegar could also contain wheat in addition to rice.

When it comes to alcoholic beverages, be aware of beer, as it is typically made from barley. Opt for gluten-free beer or explore other gluten-free options like wine or spirits.

This anecdote concerning Karen's medication can be related to. Mishap Karen, a sufferer of celiac disease, went to the drugstore to get her prescription as directed. She specifically mentioned her gluten-free requirement to the pharmacist, who assured her that the medication was safe. However, when Karen received her medication and read the label more closely, she discovered that it contained gluten.

Karen couldn't help but find the situation ironic. She jokingly remarked, "I'm trying to heal my body, not aggravate my gluten antibodies!" She immediately contacted her doctor and pharmacist to rectify the situation. From then on, Karen made it a point to double-check every medication and supplement to avoid any gluten-related mishaps.

Let's look at a story about John's Brewing Blunder. John, a gluten-free beer enthusiast, decided to try his hand at brewing his own gluten-free beer at home. He meticulously researched recipes and sourced all the necessary ingredients, excited to create his own delicious brew.

However, during the brewing process, John accidentally mixed up the ingredients and unknowingly added regular barley malt instead of gluten-free malt. The result? A beer that definitely wasn't gluten-free. When he discovered his mistake, John couldn't help but laugh at his brewing blunder.

John shared his hilarious experience with fellow gluten-free beer lovers, cautioning them to always double-check ingredients and labels. It became a running joke among his friends, and they affectionately referred to his unintentional creation as "John's Not-So-Gluten-Free Brew."

Living well and gluten-free goes beyond just following a diet. It's about embracing the adventure, finding humor in the mishaps, and savoring the joys of delicious gluten-free food. By crafting a well-balanced diet, exploring alternative grains and flours, employing innovative cooking techniques, and being mindful of hidden sources of gluten, you can lead a vibrant and enjoyable gluten-free lifestyle. Remember, relatability, humor, and friendliness make the journey more relatable, informative, and fun.

Chapter 3:

Health and Wellness on a Gluten-Free Path

Nutrition has an essential role in a gluten-free diet, and it's important to monitor deficiencies to support overall health. In this chapter, we will delve into the crucial role that nutrition plays in supporting a gluten-free diet and overall health. By understanding the connection between gluten and our well-being, managing nutrient deficiencies commonly associated with gluten-free diets, debunking gluten-related misconceptions, and embracing an active and healthy lifestyle, we can pave the way for a fulfilling and sustainable gluten-free journey.

Understanding the Connection Between Gluten and Overall Health

The key to embarking on a gluten-free path lies in understanding the connection between gluten and overall health. A gluten-free diet is essential for people with celiac disease in order to reduce inflammation and control the symptoms of the condition. Gluten consumption causes an immunological reaction that damages the small intestine and results in the autoimmune illness known as celiac disease, which manifests as a variety of symptoms.

Celiac disease, an autoimmune disorder, has a significant global impact, affecting around 1% of the population across the world (Jackson et al., 2011). The condition necessitates adherence to a rigorous gluten-free diet as the sole effective treatment. Gluten triggers an intense immune response in people with celiac disease, who then get a rash on their sensitive intestinal lining.

This persistent immune response causes substantial damage, impeding the absorption of vital nutrients. As a result, patients experience a number of unpleasant symptoms, including fatigue, bloating, and abdominal pain. Untreated celiac disease can have substantial long-term effects, making early diagnosis and dietary management essential (Harvard Health Publishing, 2017).

It is important to note that gluten can also affect individuals who are gluten-sensitive, who experience symptoms such as bloating, diarrhea, or abdominal pain when they consume gluten. When consuming gluten, people who do not have celiac disease or a wheat allergy may feel unpleasant symptoms.

This condition is known as non-celiac gluten sensitivity. While the precise cause of gluten sensitivity is unknown, it is thought to be caused by a unique immunological response or sensitivity to gluten.

Beyond celiac disease and gluten sensitivity, gluten has also been linked to a number of other health issues. It has also been connected to conditions that affect the digestive system, such as gluten ataxia, inflammatory bowel disease, and irritable bowel syndrome (IBS). Furthermore, some studies have explored potential connections between gluten and mental health issues such as depression, anxiety, and schizophrenia (Jackson et al., 2011).

While it is evident that individuals diagnosed with celiac disease, gluten sensitivity, or related health conditions must strictly avoid gluten, the potential benefits of a gluten-free diet for those without intolerance remain uncertain. For individuals not affected by these conditions, embracing a gluten-free lifestyle may not yield significant health advantages. Nonetheless, it is important to acknowledge that adhering to a gluten-free diet can indirectly foster positive alterations in eating patterns.

By encouraging the selection of whole, unprocessed foods and promoting the consumption of fruits, vegetables, and alternative grains, it can contribute to overall dietary improvements and a healthier lifestyle. Such dietary changes may increase nutrient intake and promote a more balanced approach to nutrition.

People can choose their diets wisely if they are aware of the relationship between gluten and general health. It is crucial to differentiate between the necessity of a gluten-free diet for those with celiac disease and gluten sensitivity and the potential implications for those without such conditions.

This chapter will delve into the nuances of the gluten-health relationship, shed light on the impact of gluten on different individuals, and provide a foundation for making well-informed decisions regarding gluten intake.

Managing Nutrient Deficiencies Commonly Associated with Gluten-Free Diets

It's necessary to consider the possibility of dietary deficits when switching to a gluten-free diet. A gluten-free diet is frequently linked to a number of nutrient deficiencies, underscoring the importance of paying close attention to maintain optimum nutrition. These deficiencies include B vitamins, vitamin A, magnesium, calcium, iron, and fiber, which are often found in wheat and other gluten-containing grains. The absence of these essential vitamins and minerals in a gluten-free diet can be a cause for concern, as they play vital roles in supporting various bodily functions.

To effectively manage these nutrient deficiencies and ensure a well-rounded approach to nutrition, individuals on a gluten-free path should prioritize a varied and nutrient-dense eating plan. By incorporating a wide range of naturally gluten-free foods, they can obtain the necessary nutrients to support their overall health and well-being.

An effective gluten-free diet must include plenty of fruits and vegetables. They offer a plentiful source of antioxidants, vitamins, and minerals that benefit general health. Colorful fruits and vegetables, such as berries, leafy greens, and citrus fruits, offer a diverse array of nutrients that support immune function, promote healthy digestion, and provide vital antioxidants to combat oxidative stress.

To make sure that the diet provides an adequate intake of necessary amino acids, lean proteins should also be included. Poultry, fish, beans, tofu, and eggs are examples of sources of lean proteins. These foods are high in protein, which helps to maintain satiety and promotes weight management. They also assist muscle growth and repair.

For the maintenance of healthy bones and teeth, dairy products or dairy substitutes that have been fortified with calcium and vitamin D are essential. Bone health depends on calcium, and vitamin D helps the body absorb calcium. Including dairy products or fortified alternatives like almond milk, soy milk, or coconut milk in the diet can help meet the recommended daily intake of these important nutrients.

Whole grains free of gluten are a great source of fiber, vitamins, and minerals. Examples include quinoa, brown rice, and millet. They provide energy, promote satiety, and support healthy digestion. These whole grains can be incorporated into meals as a side dish, used in salads, or included in gluten-free baking recipes.

While managing nutrient deficiencies is a crucial aspect of a gluten-free diet, it is also important to consider the individual's unique needs, and potential funny stories or experiences shared by people with celiac disease can help lighten the mood and provide relatability. Living with celiac disease often involves navigating social situations where gluten-containing foods are prevalent. Many individuals have encountered humorous situations where they mistakenly consumed gluten due to misunderstandings or mislabeled foods.

One story shared by a person with celiac disease involves attending a family gathering where a relative proudly prepared a gluten-free cake. Excitedly taking a bite, the individual soon realized that the cake was not gluten-free at all. It turned out that the relative had misunderstood the concept of gluten and used a gluten-containing flour substitute instead. Despite the unintentional mishap, everyone had a good laugh, and the relatives learned more about gluten-free ingredients.

Debunking Gluten-Related Misconceptions in Relation to Weight Loss and Gain

One prevalent misconception surrounding gluten is its association with weight gain or interference with weight loss. Many individuals believe that removing gluten from their diet will automatically lead to shedding pounds or that consuming gluten will cause them to gain weight. However, contrary to popular belief, there is no scientific evidence to suggest that gluten itself contributes to weight gain or interferes with weight loss in any meaningful way.

The weight loss often experienced by individuals who avoid gluten is primarily due to a reduction in overall carbohydrate consumption. Many foods high in carbohydrates, including bread, pasta, and baked products, contain gluten. When individuals eliminate these gluten-containing foods, they inadvertently reduce their carbohydrate intake, which can lead to weight loss. However, it is important to note that this weight loss is a result of the reduced calorie intake and not specifically because of the absence of gluten.

It is crucial to stress that a gluten-free diet is not necessarily better for you or more effective at helping you lose weight than one that contains gluten. Weight management is a complex process that depends on various factors, including overall calorie balance, nutrient composition, and individual differences. A gluten-free diet alone, without taking into account other dietary and lifestyle factors, is not a surefire way to lose weight.

The key to healthy weight management lies in adopting a balanced diet that includes a variety of nutrient-dense foods, regardless of gluten content. It is crucial to concentrate on including fresh produce, lean meats, and healthy grains in every meal. These meals offer the vital vitamins, minerals, and nutrients required for optimum health and well-being. By creating a well-rounded and nutritious eating plan, individuals can support their weight management goals while ensuring they meet their body's nutritional needs.

While debunking misconceptions, it's always interesting to hear funny stories about people's experiences with celiac disease. Living with celiac disease can present unique challenges, and sometimes humorous situations arise. For instance, imagine a person with celiac disease attending a social gathering where everyone is enjoying a delicious buffet. This person carefully asks about gluten-free options, and the host points out a plate of sandwiches labeled "gluten-free." Excitedly, the individual takes a bite, only to discover that the bread is far from gluten-free, resulting in an awkward moment of realization. These stories highlight the importance of communication, education, and awareness regarding gluten-free options, even in seemingly well-intentioned settings.

Embracing an Active and Healthy Lifestyle Alongside a Gluten-Free Regimen

In addition to focusing on nutrition, incorporating an active and healthy lifestyle is paramount for supporting overall health and well-being on a gluten-free path. Regular exercise has a host of advantages beyond just helping you lose weight. Exercise promotes cardiovascular health, increases energy, and improves mental health in addition to assisting in maintaining a healthy weight. The best part is that individuals can tailor their physical activities to their personal preferences and seamlessly integrate them into their daily routines.

Everyone can discover an activity they like because there is such a huge variety to select from. Walking is a straightforward activity that may be performed anywhere, at any time. It doesn't call for any specialized equipment and might be a terrific way to begin the journey toward an active lifestyle. Another well-liked option is running, which can be done either outside or on a treadmill, and gives the heart and lungs a cardiovascular workout.

Cycling offers a low-impact option that engages the leg muscles while exploring scenic routes. Swimming is a fantastic full-body exercise that is gentle on the joints, making it suitable for individuals of all fitness levels. Strength training, whether using free weights, resistance bands, or bodyweight exercises, helps build muscle strength and improves overall body composition.

When pursuing an active lifestyle, it is crucial to prioritize sufficient sleep and stress management. Although it is frequently overlooked, getting enough sleep is crucial for maintaining overall health. The body rejuvenates and restores itself while you sleep, supporting your best physical and mental health.

Getting enough restful sleep enables individuals to have the energy and vitality needed to engage in regular exercise and maintain a gluten-free regimen successfully. To benefit from appropriate rest, it is advised to strive for 7–9 hours of sleep per night.

The ability to regulate stress is essential for general health. Chronic stress can have detrimental effects on health, including compromising the immune system, impairing digestion, and contributing to mental health issues. It is crucial to find effective techniques to manage stress and incorporate them into daily routines. Practices such as meditation, deep breathing exercises, or engaging in enjoyable activities like reading, listening to music, or spending time in nature can significantly reduce stress levels and promote a sense of calm and balance.

Hydration is another vital aspect of maintaining an active and healthy lifestyle. Water is required for healthy biological activities like digestion, vitamin absorption, and cleansing. Staying hydrated throughout the day supports these vital functions and ensures the body operates efficiently.

It is advised to hydrate well and pay attention to the body's thirst cues. Adequate hydration can also help maintain energy levels and prevent dehydration-related fatigue during physical activities.

By embracing an active and healthy lifestyle alongside a gluten-free regimen, individuals can experience a synergistic effect on their overall well-being. Engaging in regular physical activity, prioritizing sufficient sleep, managing stress effectively, and staying hydrated all contribute to supporting the body's optimal functioning. Furthermore, the combination of an active lifestyle and a gluten-free diet promotes a holistic approach to health, addressing both physical and dietary needs.

Remember to consult with healthcare professionals or fitness experts to tailor an exercise routine that suits your individual needs and abilities. It is essential to listen to the body, set realistic goals, and gradually increase activity levels to avoid injury or burnout. By finding joy and fulfillment in an active lifestyle alongside gluten-free choices, individuals can enhance their well-being, cultivate healthy habits, and embark on a sustainable journey toward overall health and vitality.

Chapter 4:

Beyond Gluten: Expanding Your Culinary Horizons

In this chapter, we break free from the notion that a gluten-free diet is restrictive or mundane. We'll ignite your culinary curiosity and take you on a flavorful trip around the world, exploring international cuisines that offer delightful gluten-free options. From mouthwatering desserts to creative recipes that will unleash your inner chef, get ready to discover a whole new world of delicious possibilities.

Exploring the World of Gluten-Free International Cuisines

When it comes to a gluten-free diet, there is a common misconception that it limits your culinary options and leaves you with a mundane and restrictive menu. But nothing could be further from the truth than that! In this section, we embark on a flavorful journey around the world, exploring international cuisines that offer a plethora of delightful gluten-free options. From Italian delicacies to Latin American temptations, Thai experiences, Middle Eastern sensations, and Indian delicacies, get ready to discover a whole new world of delicious possibilities.

Italian Delights

Italian cuisine is renowned for its use of wheat-based pasta and bread. But there are also many delicious gluten-free options available in Italy. Risotto, made with arborio rice, becomes a creamy and comforting dish that can be customized with various ingredients like vegetables, seafood, or cheese. Polenta, crafted from cornmeal, is another Italian staple that can be transformed into delectable dishes, such as creamy polenta with mushroom ragout or crispy polenta fries. With the right ingredients and techniques, Italian cuisine can be a haven for gluten-free food lovers.

Latin American Temptations

Latin American cuisine is vibrant, diverse, and packed with gluten-free options. From the flavorful beans and corn-based soft tortillas and tortilla chips to an array of rice dishes like arroz con pollo (chicken with rice), Latin American cuisine provides a multitude of gluten-free delights. Tacos, enchiladas, and tamales can easily be made gluten-free with corn tortillas, while dishes like ceviche, guacamole, and grilled meats offer fresh and zesty flavors. Don't forget to indulge in the popular Brazilian cheese bread, Po de Queijo, made with tapioca flour and cheese, which is naturally gluten-free and incredibly addictive.

Thai Experiences

Thai cuisine is known for its bold and aromatic flavors, and it also happens to be naturally gluten-free. Rice takes center stage in Thai cuisine, making dishes like fragrant jasmine rice, pineapple fried rice, and coconut rice a staple. Rice noodles are another gluten-free alternative that can be enjoyed in classic Thai dishes like pad thai or spicy tom yum soup. Curry dishes thickened with creamy coconut milk, such as green curry or massaman curry, offer a symphony of flavors that will transport you to the bustling streets of Thailand. Thai food is a gluten-free lover's heaven with its profusion of fresh herbs, spices, and colorful flavors.

Middle Eastern Sensations

Middle Eastern cuisine is a treasure trove of gluten-free options. Chickpeas and broad beans are transformed into delicious dips like hummus and baba ganoush, which can be enjoyed with gluten-free pita bread or fresh vegetables. The aromatic spices and flavors of the region come alive in dishes like falafel, which are spiced and fried chickpea balls that are gluten-free and incredibly satisfying. Grilled meats, kebabs, and rice-based dishes like mujadara (rice and lentils) or mansaf (Jordanian lamb and yogurt rice) offer a feast for the senses. Middle Eastern cuisine celebrates bold flavors and gluten-free ingredients, making it a must-try for those on a gluten-free journey.

Indian Delicacies

Indian cuisine is as diverse as its culture, and it offers a plethora of gluten-free delights. From street food favorites to elaborate curries, Indian cuisine is a playground of flavors and textures. Savory snacks like tikkas (grilled meat or vegetable skewers) and pakoras (fried fritters) are often gluten-free and bursting with aromatic spices. South Indian cuisine features dishes like dosas (thin rice and lentil crepes) and idlis (steamed rice cakes), which are naturally gluten-free and can be enjoyed with flavorful chutneys and sambar. North Indian cuisine boasts gluten-free options like butter chicken, biryani (spiced rice dishes), and dal (lentil curries). With its rich heritage and diverse regional specialties, Indian cuisine provides a world of gluten-free delicacies.

Indulging in Delicious Gluten-Free Desserts and Treats

When it comes to gluten-free desserts, the possibilities are endless. The days of giving up delectable delicacies to follow a gluten-free diet are long gone. You can sate your desire for sweets without sacrificing flavor using cutting-edge ingredients and inventive cooking methods. From classic favorites to inventive confections and dairy-free delights, let's explore the world of gluten-free desserts and treats.

Sweet Temptations

Desserts free of gluten are available in a wide range of sizes and shapes to suit different tastes and dietary requirements. Indulge in a variety of gluten-free cakes, cookies, brownies, pies, puddings, and pavlovas that will satisfy your sweet cravings. From decadent flourless chocolate cake to fruity and refreshing sorbets, the world of gluten-free desserts offers a delightful array of options. With gluten-free flour blends, alternative grains like almond flour or coconut flour, and natural sweeteners like maple syrup or honey, you can recreate your favorite desserts in a gluten-free version.

Creative Confections

Unleash your inner pastry chef and let your creativity shine with inventive gluten-free recipes. Martha Stewart's coconut-pecan tart, for example, features an easy press-in crust made from shredded coconut and almond flour. This gluten-free tart is a testament to the fact that gluten-free baking can be just as delicious and impressive as traditional baking. Experiment with different flours, like buckwheat or quinoa flour, to add depth of flavor and texture to your creations. From fruit galettes to layered mousse cakes, gluten-free baking opens up a world of possibilities for the adventurous home cook.

Dairy-Free Delights

For those who follow a gluten-free and dairy-free diet, there are plenty of options to satisfy their dessert cravings. It is now simpler than ever to enjoy delectable dairy-free foods thanks to the growth of plant-based substitutes. Discover the realm of gluten-free and dairy-free dessert recipes, such as vegan key lime pie, chocolate-cherry fudge torte with cherry sorbet, vegan millionaire's shortbread, berry nice cream cake, and vegan lemon cheesecake. With ingredients like coconut milk, almond milk, and dairy-free chocolate, you can create creamy and indulgent desserts that are free from both gluten and dairy.

Unleashing Your Inner Chef with Creative Gluten-Free Recipes

Cooking gluten-free doesn't have to be complicated or boring. In fact, it might be a fascinating chance to experiment with new foods, tastes, and methods. Whether you're a seasoned chef or a beginner in the kitchen, there are plenty of resources available to help you create delicious and satisfying gluten-free meals. Embrace your inner chef as we explore the world of gluten-free cooking.

Whole Foods Inspiration

Celebrate the beauty of whole foods and enjoy easy and flavorful gluten-free meals. Downshiftology, a popular food blog, offers a comprehensive guide featuring over 40 gluten-free recipes that celebrate fresh, nourishing ingredients. By focusing on whole foods like vegetables, fruits, lean proteins, and gluten-free grains like quinoa or brown rice, these recipes provide a wide array of options for creating satisfying and wholesome meals. From vibrant and hearty salads bursting with flavor to grain-free bowls packed with nutrients and delicious stir-fries that showcase the natural colors and textures of fresh ingredients, Downshiftology's guide proves that gluten-free cooking can be both nourishing and delicious. Whether you're a seasoned gluten-free cook or just starting your gluten-free journey, exploring the world of whole foods will introduce you to new and exciting flavors while providing the nourishment your body deserves. With Downshiftology's guide, you can discover new favorites that will become staples in your gluten-free repertoire.

Home Cook Favorites

Sometimes the best recipes come from fellow home cooks who have perfected their gluten-free creations. Allrecipes, a popular online recipe community, offers a vast collection of over 1,430 gluten-free recipes contributed by home cooks from around the world. Browse through the extensive collection, read helpful reviews and insights, and find inspiration for your next gluten-free meal. Whether you're in the mood for comforting casseroles, flavorful soups, or delightful desserts, you'll find a treasure trove of recipes to suit your taste and dietary needs.

Gourmet Gluten-Free

If you're looking to elevate your gluten-free cooking and indulge in gourmet dishes, look no further than Bon Appétit's collection of 77 gluten-free recipes. From satisfying breakfast options like gluten-free pancakes to mouthwatering desserts like flourless chocolate cake, these recipes combine elegance and flavor. Discover the world of gluten-free gourmet cooking and wow your loved ones with home-cooked meals that rival those served in restaurants.

Taste of Home

Taste of Home, a cherished magazine and website that celebrates the joy of home cooking, has curated a collection of 50 exceptional gluten-free recipes. This compilation covers all aspects of gluten-free cooking, from delectable desserts to crowd-pleasing dinners and irresistible bread recipes. With Taste of Home, you can savor the familiar and comforting flavors that evoke the warmth and nostalgia of home.

Indulge in the sweet aromas of freshly baked cinnamon rolls, whose soft and fluffy texture is delightfully gluten-free. Experience the satisfaction of biting into a perfectly breaded and golden chicken Parmesan without compromising your dietary needs. And for those moments when you crave a side of warm, cheesy garlic bread to accompany your meal, Taste of Home has you covered with a gluten-free version that delivers the same mouthwatering flavors.

The recipes featured in Taste of Home's gluten-free collection have been tested and approved by home cooks who understand the importance of delicious gluten-free options. With their seal of approval, you can trust that each recipe has been crafted with care and precision to ensure both taste and dietary compliance.

Whether you're a gluten-free veteran or embarking on a new culinary journey, Taste of Home's gluten-free recipes provide a gateway to discovering new favorites and enjoying the comforting taste of home. With their dedication to quality and the shared experiences of a vibrant cooking community, Taste of Home brings the joys of home cooking to the gluten-free table.

Funny Stories and Experiences from Others Living Gluten-Free

Living a gluten-free lifestyle can sometimes lead to amusing and unexpected situations. Let's take a lighthearted look at some funny stories and experiences shared by individuals who follow a gluten-free diet.

Popcorn Puzzlement: One Reddit user shared a comical encounter at the movies when they asked the person working behind the counter if the popcorn was gluten-free. I don't know, do you want to sample it and see?" was the bewildered employee's reply. This amusing response highlights the lack of awareness about gluten-free options in unexpected places. It's a reminder that even seemingly simple questions can lead to amusing responses and highlight the need for education and awareness regarding gluten-free ingredients.

Cheese Confusion: In a restaurant setting, a gluten-free diner ordered a seasonal steak dish that came with a wedge of Stilton cheese. Concerned about the base of the cheese, she called over the waiter for clarification. To her surprise, the waiter confidently informed her that the cheese was made out of graham crackers. When she questioned him about the ingredients of graham crackers, he hilariously replied, "Grahams?" This story emphasizes the need for education and awareness regarding gluten-free ingredients. Additionally, it emphasizes how crucial good communication is when trying to accommodate dietary restrictions.

Misguided Mix-Up: Another Reddit user shared a humorous incident at a social gathering. The user, who follows a gluten-free diet, attended a potluck where someone brought a dish labeled "gluten-free lasagna." Excitedly, the user took a generous portion of the dish, only to discover that it was, in fact, regular lasagna and not gluten-free as claimed. This mishap highlights the importance of clear labeling and communication when it comes to accommodating dietary restrictions. It reminds us that assumptions can lead to funny and unexpected situations.

These funny stories remind us that living gluten-free can sometimes lead to amusing and unexpected situations.

While they bring a smile to our faces, they also serve as a reminder of the need for awareness, understanding, and clear communication in culinary settings. Living gluten-free doesn't have to be dull or restrictive, and by embracing international cuisines, indulging in delicious desserts, exploring creative recipes, and sharing lighthearted stories, we can break free from the notion that a gluten-free diet is anything less than flavorful and enjoyable.

Conclusion

Embracing a gluten-free lifestyle goes beyond dietary restrictions, offering individuals a transformative experience that positively impacts their health and overall well-being. By adopting a gluten-free diet, individuals can experience improvements in their physical and mental health, leading to a deeper appreciation for the choices they make to prioritize their well-being. This lifestyle shift opens doors to a world of possibilities, empowering individuals to make informed decisions that positively impact various aspects of their lives.

From exploring new culinary creations and connecting with a supportive gluten-free community to enjoying an expanding market of gluten-free products and increased accessibility in dining establishments, individuals can fully embrace the benefits of a gluten-free lifestyle. By reflecting on the positive impact of their choices, individuals can enhance their overall quality of life and find fulfillment in the journey of gluten-free living.

The decision to embrace a gluten-free lifestyle requires self-acceptance and resilience. It is a process that involves understanding and acknowledging one's dietary needs, which can initially feel overwhelming and challenging. When individuals first discover that they need to adopt a gluten-free diet, they may need to reassess their eating habits, educate themselves about gluten-free ingredients, and find suitable alternatives for their favorite foods.

However, through this journey, individuals develop a sense of self-acceptance. They learn to embrace their unique dietary requirements, accepting that their health and well-being are of utmost importance. This process of self-acceptance is a powerful step towards self-empowerment and serves as a catalyst for personal growth.

In addition to personal growth, the availability of resources and support within the gluten-free community plays a significant role in navigating the gluten-free adventure. Online platforms, cookbooks, support groups, and forums provide a wealth of information and guidance. These resources offer practical tips for grocery shopping, meal planning, and cooking while also sharing experiences and stories from individuals who have successfully embraced a gluten-free lifestyle. People might gain inspiration, support, and reassurance by connecting with others who are traveling along similar paths. They recognize that there is a supporting group who shares their struggles and victories, and that they are not alone. The shift to a gluten-free lifestyle is made easier and more tolerable by this feeling of community and friendship.

The chance to experiment with countless recipes and culinary creations is one of the most exciting benefits of adopting a gluten-free lifestyle. With the growing awareness of gluten-free dietary needs, there is an abundance of resources available to individuals looking to experiment in the kitchen. From traditional dishes adapted to be gluten-free to innovative and creative recipes specifically designed for those with dietary restrictions, the possibilities are endless.

Individuals can find gluten-free versions of their favorite dishes, such as pizza, pasta, and baked goods, allowing them to continue enjoying the flavors they love. Moreover, they can discover new flavors and ingredients that they may not have previously considered. The gluten-free journey invites individuals to indulge their culinary curiosity and create delightful meals that are both delicious and nourishing.

The market for gluten-free products is expanding rapidly, driven by the increasing demand for gluten-free alternatives. Food businesses are starting to realize how important it is to accommodate those who have celiac disease or gluten allergies. This growing market not only ensures a wider selection of gluten-free products on store shelves, but also encourages innovation and improved quality. Food manufacturers are constantly developing new gluten-free options, from bread and pasta to snacks and desserts.

They are experimenting with different gluten-free flours, grains, and ingredients to create products that are both safe and satisfying for individuals following a gluten-free lifestyle. As the market continues to grow, individuals can expect a greater variety of gluten-free options, making it easier to find suitable alternatives for their favorite foods and enjoy a diverse and satisfying diet.

Every day, it becomes increasingly easier to find places to eat gluten-free outside of the home. Restaurants, cafés, and food establishments are becoming more aware of the need to accommodate individuals with gluten sensitivities or celiac disease. Many establishments now offer dedicated gluten-free menus or clearly label gluten-free options, making dining out a more enjoyable experience for those following a gluten-free lifestyle.

This increased accessibility not only provides convenience, but also fosters a sense of inclusivity and empowerment. Individuals no longer have to worry about being limited to certain types of cuisine or feeling left out during social gatherings. They can confidently navigate menus, ask questions about ingredients, and choose dishes that align with their dietary needs. This progress in the food industry not only reflects the growing demand for gluten-free options, but also signifies a shift towards a more inclusive and accommodating dining culture.

Although adopting a gluten-free lifestyle has many advantages, it is crucial to be aware of potential nutritional shortages and get regular exercise. A gluten-free diet, if not properly balanced, may lack certain nutrients, such as fiber, B vitamins, and iron. This is because many gluten-containing grains, such as wheat, barley, and rye, are significant sources of these nutrients. To ensure optimal nutrition, it is important to prioritize a well-rounded and varied diet that incorporates a wide range of gluten-free whole foods.

Foods like fruits, vegetables, lean proteins, and gluten-free grains like quinoa, rice, and amaranth help make up for any nutrients that may be missing from a gluten-free diet. Additionally, consulting with a healthcare professional or registered dietitian who specializes in gluten-free nutrition can provide valuable guidance in ensuring optimal nutrition while adhering to a gluten-free lifestyle.

Exercise on a regular basis is essential for preserving general health and well-being, along with proper nutrition. Exercise not only supports cardiovascular fitness and muscular strength, but also contributes to mental well-being and stress reduction. By incorporating physical activity into daily routines, individuals can enhance their gluten-free journey and promote a balanced and active lifestyle. Finding pleasurable, long-lasting activities is crucial for achieving the best possible health outcomes since they improve the likelihood of sustained participation.

Whether it's going for a walk, practicing yoga, participating in sports, or joining fitness classes, finding activities that bring joy and fulfillment can make the gluten-free journey even more rewarding. Regular exercise also aids in weight management and improves digestion, further contributing to the overall well-being of individuals embracing a gluten-free lifestyle.

References

Anderson, J. (2020, July 10). *How to dine out gluten-free at restaurants that serve global cuisine.* Verywell Fit. https://www.verywellfit.com/dining-gluten-free-at-ethnic-restaurants-562723

Bryan , L. (2021, March 8). *40+ best gluten-free recipes.* Downshiftology. https://downshiftology.com/best-gluten-free-recipes/

Celiac disease. (2021, August 10). Mayo Clinic. https://www.mayoclinic.org/diseases-conditions/celiac-disease/symptoms-causes/syc-20352220

Cleveland Clinic. (2023, May 3). *Surprising foods that contain gluten.* https://health.clevelandclinic.org/what-foods-have-gluten/

Gluten: A benefit or harm to the body? (2018, April 20). Harvard School of Public Health. https://www.hsph.harvard.edu/nutritionsource/gluten/

Gluten-free diet. (2021, December 11). Mayo Clinic. https://www.mayoclinic.org/healthy-lifestyle/nutrition-and-healthy-eating/in-depth/gluten-free-diet/art-20048530

Gorin, A. (2018, August 29*). Gluten myths and facts to know.* Everyday Health. https://www.everydayhealth.com/diet-nutrition/diet/gluten-myths-facts-know/

Hansen, M. (2020, May 9). *The complete guide to eating out gluten-free.* Wheatless Wanderlust. https://wheatlesswanderlust.com/eating-out-gluten-free-dining/

Harvard Health Publishing. (2017, April 12). *Ditch the Gluten, Improve Your Health?* Harvard Health; Harvard Health. https://www.health.harvard.edu/staying-healthy/ditch-the-gluten-improve-your-health

Healthy weight gain in celiac disease. (2021). GIG. https://gluten.org/wp-content/uploads/2021/08/EDU_Healthy-weight-gain.pdf

Jackson, J. R., Eaton, W. W., Cascella, N. G., Fasano, A., & Kelly, D. L. (2011). Neurologic and Psychiatric Manifestations of Celiac Disease and Gluten Sensitivity. *Psychiatric Quarterly, 83*(1), 91–102. https://doi.org/10.1007/s11126-011-9186-y

Kim, F. (2022, December 20). *25 supremely delicious gluten-free dessert recipes.* Martha Stewart. https://www.marthastewart.com/1504289/gluten-free-desserts

Kubala, J. (2019, March 6). *Is gluten bad for you? A critical look.* Healthline.

https://www.healthline.com/nutrition/is-gluten-bad#intolerance

Nardone, S. (n.d.). *Why cacao butter should be your valentine*. Food Network. https://www.foodnetwork.com/healthyeats/recipes/2016/02/why-cacao-butter-should-be-your-valentine

Ratner, A. (2019, February 26). *Misconceptions about the gluten-free diet*. Gluten-Free Living. https://www.glutenfreeliving.com/gluten-free/dispelling-myths/misconceptions-about-the-gluten-free-diet/

Restaurant dining: Seven tips for staying gluten-free. (2019, October 18). Gluten Intolerance Group. https://gluten.org/2019/10/18/restaurant-dining-seven-tips-for-staying-gluten-free/

35+ alternative gluten-free grains and flour substitutes. (2022, January). GIG. https://gluten.org/2019/10/17/gluten-free-grains/

2023 trends and opportunities in gluten-free – article. (2023, February 17). New Hope Network. https://www.newhope.com/products-and-trends/2023-trends-and-opportunities-gluten-free-article